DEFIANT CHILDREN

When your Kid isn't just Difficult

by

Brittany Forrester

Brittany Forrester© Copyright 2021 - All rights reserved.

The content contained within this book may not be reproduced, duplicated, or transmitted without direct written permission from the author or the publisher.

Under no circumstances will any blame or legal responsibility be held against the publisher, or author, for any damages, reparation, or monetary loss due to the information contained within this book. Either directly or indirectly.

Legal Notice:

This book is copyright protected. This book is only for personal use. You cannot amend, distribute, sell, use, quote, or paraphrase any part, or the content within this book, without the consent of the author or publisher.

Disclaimer Notice:

Please note the information contained within this document is for educational and entertainment purposes only. All effort has been executed to present accurate, up-to-date, and reliable, complete information. No warranties of any kind are declared or implied. Readers acknowledge that the author is not engaging in the rendering of legal, financial, medical, or professional advice. The content within this book has been derived from various sources. Please consult a licensed professional before attempting any techniques outlined in this book.

By reading this document, the reader agrees that under no circumstances is the author responsible for any losses, direct or indirect, which are incurred as a result of the use of the information contained within this document, including, but not limited to, — errors, omissions, or inaccuracies.

Table of Contents

What is Oppositional Defiant Disorder..................5
Associations with ODD....................................8
Predicting ODD..9
Social Adversity..16
Diagnostic Considerations...............................17
Social maladjustment as Oppositional Defiant Disorder
....21
Emotions..24
ETIOLOGY AND RISK FACTORS.....................30
    Genetics...30
    Age of onset..31
    Temperament..31
    Peer influences...32
    Callous and unemotional traits...................32
    Neighborhoods...33
    Family factors..33
    Models of family influences.......................34
ODD within the School Setting.........................35
Family Approach to School-Based Intervention....37
Treatment Approaches to Oppositional Defiant Disorder..39
Sex differences in oppositional defiant disorder....47
Age differences in oppositional defiant disorder...50
Culture differences in oppositional defiant disorder..53

Oppositional Defiant Disorder in Adolescents...........54
Parental approach..63
Advice for parenting ODD..66
Diet..69
Parental Problem solving to manage ODD.................71
ODD, autism, and ADHD...73
Conclusions..77

What is Oppositional Defiant Disorder

Oppositional defiant disorder (ODD) is the most common clinical disorder in children and adolescents, with a prevalence of 6.5 % in adolescents. Children and adolescents with ODD struggle with respecting authority and often display animosity, noncompliance, and negativity towards those in authority. Conduct disorder (CD), has a prevalence of 2.2 % in adolescents but is considered to have more severe behavioral symptoms than ODD. Children and adolescents with CD typically behave in ways that disrespect social norms and the rights of others, demonstrating aggression towards people, animals, and property, as well as engaging in deceit.

A diagnosis of CD often follows a previous diagnosis of ODD in early childhood. Earlier onset of CD/ODD is correlated with the development of antisocial personality disorder, substance-related disorders, increased rates of drug use (tobacco and alcohol), mood disorders, anxiety disorders, somatoform disorders, and higher accident rates. Additionally, CD/ODD diagnoses are often comorbid with attention-deficit/hyperactivity disorder (ADHD) diagnoses. ADHD is a neurological disorder involving inattentiveness and/or hyperactive and impulsive behaviors that appear before the age of 12 years. Until recently, these three disorders were classified together as disruptive behavior disorders, in the Diagnostic and Statistical Manual of Mental Disorders, and are still quite commonly referred to as externalizing disorders.

They also share several distinct neurological and physiological characteristics including executive functioning deficits and hypo-responsivity to stressors. An individual who has been diagnosed with CD/ODD has a prognosis for low levels of success in school settings and later employment success. In considering treatment for individuals diagnosed with CD and/or ODD, the impact on society increases as the child ages, and the resources required increase exponentially.

It has been estimated that by the time children with CD reach 28 years of age, they access 10 times the amount of public/government-funded services as those without CD — totaling an estimated US$140,000 in additional services for each individual with CD. Research suggests that the most effective treatments for children with CD/ODD focus not on symptomology, but on factors, such as parenting, that promote the development of these disorders. Some researchers have made the claim that intra-familial social processes and familial risk factors are of primary importance when considering CD/ODD development. Carr's wide-ranging review reported that family-based interventions are effective for externalizing behavior problems. Attachment theory provides a sound theoretical framework for the development of CD/ODD in consideration of these intra-familial social processes and familial risk factors.

Insecure attachments produce deficits in effective functioning — precisely empathetic functioning and modulation of unpleasant emotional states — they create an ideal risk factor for the development of CD/ODD. Attachment insecurity will not on its lead to conduct disorder.

Associations with ODD

Though emotion socialization and emotion regulation were the focus of the present study, Psychological analyses demonstrate that children's lability and ADHD symptoms also play a role in children's ODD symptoms. Particularly, pre-treatment lability and ADHD symptoms were linked to post-treatment ODD symptoms. These elements are consistent with the clinical presentation of ODD, in that it is highly comorbid with ADHD and is characterized by inflexible emotional expression. These findings indicate that children's emotional lability and other externalizing behaviors play a role in children's treatment response, in that there are poorer treatment outcomes for children diagnosed with ADHD and those who are more emotionally volatile.

Predicting ODD

Some people ask if the ODD is predictable, well psychologists agree about some peculiarities that affect children's emotional life and behavior in general. ODD has concurrently, and its association with difficulties in adulthood, investigations into the potential antecedents to its onset are important for developing both preventative and acute treatments. Research has shown that disruptive behavior disorders are more prevalent in boys and there may be gender differences in the processes by which varying factors convey the risk of ODD. Well documented risk factors for the development of anti-social behavior (ASB) and DBDs include socioeconomic adversity, maladaptive parental behavior such as substance abuse, and family instability. Further recent research has aimed to explore the mechanisms by which these risk factors may convey negative effects on child disruptive behavior. However, less is known about the etiology of ODD independent of CD.

This book aims to investigate the contribution of maternal anger, in the postpartum period, as a mediator in the relationship between maternal depression (an internalizing disorder) and the development of ODD (an externalizing disorder in young children, while accounting for other related risk factors. Each antecedent of interest is explored below.

Maternal depression has been consistently associated with the onset of expression and the postnatal period. Depression is often an episodic and recurrent disorder; a history of depression is a significant predictor of perinatal depression, and women with perinatal depression are at greater risk of experiencing subsequent episodes of depression, both within future pregnancies and postnatal, and outside of the perinatal period. However, despite the chronic nature of depression, there is some evidence that the timing of depressive episodes may have a differential effect on kid outcome. Postpartum depression appears to convey a unique problem for deficits in cognitive development and depression across the perinatal period is important in the prediction of offspring emotional development.

However, the evidence to date on children's emotional development is based on dimensional measures of problems, none of the studies have used standardized diagnostic interviews to determine clinically significant externalizing mental health problems in children.

Also, few have measured maternal depression by clinical interview; the majority have used a self-reported questionnaire-based continuous measure of maternal depression. Furthermore, significant associations between maternal depression and externalizing problems in the child may be related to attribution biases of the informant, rather than an objective association between the two concepts. Another factor could be the Maternal Anger.

Is hypothesized that maternal anger will be positively related to child ODD, and a diagnosis that has been characterized by anger. In one theory of emotional development,

Psychologists suggest that one of the fundamental ways in which propensities to emotions develop in children is through observational learning, or their parents' expression of emotion in the home. Studies show that anger, a component of conflict, may play a significant role in the association between marital conflict and child problems; overt and intense displays of anger and aggression by parents show more association with child psychopathology than ratings of either covert tension in the relationship or a lack of conflict resolution.

Depression is considered; one such way in which maternal depression may manifest and convey risk for externalizing disorders in children, such as ODD, is through maternal anger. Higher levels of anger in individuals with depression compared to those who are well have been consistently shown.

One such theory for the common heightened frequency between depression and anger is that they are both considered to be responses to the blocking of a positive reinforcer; depression/sadness is the passive response resulting from helplessness to gain the reinforcer, and anger is a motivating response that rallies an individual to gain the reinforce, when such action is possible. Even if, Freud theorized that depression was anger turned inward, it may be the case, however, that individuals move between the two emotions, meeting criteria for depression whilst also experiencing anger alongside. Indeed, anger has been associated with the common, yet under-recognized, symptom of irritability in major depression.

The co-occurrence of depression and anger continues in the parental context. Women with high anger describe more negative experiences with the entry to parenthood compared to women with low anger.

Depression is thought to manifest in the mother-infant relationship as high levels of intrusive and/or withdrawn behaviors, with the former style associated with anger and irritation directed at the infant. Parental behavior characterized by anger and aggression has been associated with increased ODD in children Together, these findings suggest that maternal anger expression may be an important avenue for investigation, both independently and in the context of depression.

In furthering the understanding of the prediction of ODD, along with other psychopathology, particular attention should be paid to the preschool years. Infants are affected by the emotional climate of the home from a young age and respond differently to anger and other emotions from very early in life. At five months of age, infants can distinguish between negative emotions, even in unfamiliar languages, and at three-months, they show varied responses to anger and other emotions in their mothers' voices.

Thus the effect of maternal anger from early infancy, a stage where maternal emotion is likely to be influencing the development of the child's emotional tendencies and later child behavior.

Babies are sensitive to the emotional climate of their environment as emotions are a crucial communicative tool at this age; infants use parents' emotions to guide their behavior in the short term, and their reactions to their parents' emotions predict their later socio-emotional development The expression of anger in maternal behavior may impact upon the development of the child's' own emotional repertoire through social learning, or by shaping their likelihood to adopt particular emotional communicative styles. Indeed, excessive anger at two years of age predicts an increased risk of psychopathology at age 5, and children with early-onset disruptive behavior problems are more likely to show poorer outcomes later in life than those who develop symptoms during adolescence.

Mothers' antisocial history is associated with their children's conduct problems. Antisocial problems are also associated with depression, both generally and in the perinatal period

Therefore, it is important to consider whether it is depressed women's antisocial history that drives the relationship between depression and/or maternal anger on ODD, and/or whether a mothers' antisocial history is related to child ODD directly. It may also be the case that a mother's already established propensity to antisocial behavior explains the relationship between maternal anger and depression in the perinatal period with later child difficulties.

Social Adversity

There is also a need to consider the complex interplay between psychological and social risk factors for childhood ODD; it may be the case that, in a demographically diverse population, social adversity moderates the relationship between the hypothesized predictors and ODD. Rates of well-known risk factors, such as maternal depression, vary across population groups. Depressed mothers are more likely to draw from socioeconomically disadvantaged backgrounds and have lower educational and teen pregnancy is a well-known risk factor for perinatal depression. Whilst high-risk samples allow for the specific study of Therefore, this book will consider whether social adversity is related to ODD directly, and/or moderates the relationship between maternal anger and ODD; it may be that maternal anger is associated with child ODD differentially, according to whether families are of particular levels of adversity.

Diagnostic Considerations

There are currently two primary symptom categories used to diagnose ODD - externalizing behavior problems and negative emotions. There are currently eight symptoms of ODD listed in the DSM-V that include:

(1) arguing with authority figures or adults;

(2) actively defying or refusing to comply with rules/requests from authority figures;

(3) deliberately annoying others;

(4) blaming others for their own mistakes or misbehaviors;

(5) prone to being touchy, irritable, or easily annoyed;

(6) easily losing temper;

(7) often being angry and resentful;

(8) has been spiteful or vindictive at least twice within the past six months.

For a diagnosis of ODD to be considered, the presence of four or more symptoms is required for at least six months. Symptoms also must present with a frequency and persistence that exceed similar behaviors in typically developing peers (i.e., contribute to significant distress and impaired social, educational, and/or occupational functioning). Further, the primary problems associated with ODD are distinct from other conditions in that they frequently violate the rights of others.

Prevalence and Course Disruptive behavior disorders such as ODD are considered to be the most prevalent childhood psychiatric conditions in need of psychological services. Though generally a high base rate condition overall, the prevalence of ODD reported across clinical studies varies widely (1% to 11%). Data from community samples suggest that its prevalence may reach as high as 15.6% in some populations.

There are also notable differences in the presentation of ODD based upon age, gender, and environmental factors. About age, ODD symptoms typically arise during preschool years and seldom present later than adolescence. Though ODD is widely believed to be influenced by individual child temperament, there are no known biological or genetic predictors specific to the disorder. Although ODD symptoms often present early, the nature and severity of these symptoms often change in adolescence and early adulthood. A distinct, developmental relationship has been established between ODD and both Conduct Disorder (CD) and depression. Reported gender differences in ODD suggest that boys meet criteria more frequently than girls. However, gender differences appear to dissipate in adolescence and beyond. While girls appear to be more at risk for later developing depression after experiencing ODD, boys show a greater proclivity for developing CD. Environmental factors known to contribute to the emergence of ODD include higher family conflict and parenting stress as well as multiple socioeconomic variables. The evidence to date suggests that ODD symptoms are most directly accounted for by families' reports of parenting stress and poorer family functioning overall.

The relation between these contextual factors and the development of ODD dates back to Gerald Patterson's descriptions of "coercive family processes." Patterson depicts a gradual development of ODD symptoms that are brought about by an interaction between a difficult child temperament and reactive, authoritarian, and inconsistent parenting. The developmental course of ODD symptoms often reveals a consistent increase in severity over time that frequently progresses to diagnoses of Conduct

Disorder (CD), depression, or other major mental health concerns. The developmental course of ODD is also frequently complicated by comorbidity with other conditions. This appears to be the rule rather than the exception with nearly 50% of all ODD cases presenting co-occurring ADHD, 40% reporting significant anxiety symptoms, and 12% being diagnosed with depression. When depression later follows childhood-onset of ODD, it is best predicted by the prominence of ODD-related negative effect. Likewise, children presenting more dominant symptoms of defiance and antagonistic behaviors frequently progress from ODD to later symptoms more representative of CD. There is an estimated correlation between the symptoms of ODD and CD, which ultimately reflects an extremely high degree of symptom comorbidity. Despite the strong evidence supporting ODD as a predictor of future behavioral and emotional problems, it remains unclear if its role is causal, prodromal, or simply a precursor to future concerns.

Social maladjustment as Oppositional Defiant Disorder

A diagnostic parallel to the term "social maladjustment" nowadays is "oppositional defiant disorder" ODD as defined below: pattern of angry/irritable mood, argumentative/defiant behavior, or vindictiveness lasting at least 6/8 months as evidenced by at least four symptoms from any of the following categories, and exhibited during interaction with at least one individual who is not a relative. It is very common for individuals with oppositional defiant disorder to show symptoms only at home and only with family members. However, the prevalence of the symptoms is an indicator of the severity of the disorder.

The criteria to recognize ODD have as said before different peculiarities. An Angry or Irritable Mood, for instance, is someone who often loses temper and is often touchy or easily annoyed, or even often angry and resentful. This argumentative/Defiant Behavior, often argues with authority figures or, for children and adolescents, with adults. Usually actively defies or refuses to comply with requests or with rules.

- Often deliberately annoys others. - Often blames others for his or her mistakes or misbehavior. At least is always vindictive, or has been spiteful or vindictive with people.

The persistence and frequency of these behaviors should be used to distinguish a behavior that is within normal limits from a symptomatic behavior. For children younger than 5/6 years old, the behavior should occur on most days for at least 6/7 months unless otherwise notes. For children 5/6 years or older, the behavior should occur at least once per week for at least 6/7months, unless otherwise notes. While these frequency criteria guide a minimal level of frequency to define symptoms, other factors should also be considered, such as whether the frequency and intensity of the behaviors are outside a range that is normative for the individuals' developmental level, gender, and culture.

The disturbance in behavior is associated with distress in the individual or others in his or her immediate social context (e.g., family, peer group, work colleagues), or it impacts negatively on social, educational, occupational, or other important areas of functioning. The behaviors do not occur exclusively during a psychotic, substance use, depressive, or bipolar disorder. Also, the criteria are not met for disruptive mood dysregulation disorder.

Emotions

Children with ODD/CD have been found to exhibit difficulties in the regulation of their own emotions the processes by which individuals influence which emotions they have, when they have them, and how they experience and express these emotions. Studies have reported that kids with aggressive and antisocial behavior used less effective or more inappropriate regulatory strategies. Besides these problems in emotion regulation, children with ODD/CD have also been found to have specific problems in affect recognition.

Self-regulation refers to "the process by which people initiate, adjust, interrupt, stop or otherwise change thoughts, feelings or actions to affect the realization of personal aims or plans or to maintain a current standard" This definition indicates that self-regulation can be a conscious process. However, even before one unconsciously acts to control emotion, thought, or behavior, regulatory processes at a neuro-biological level already take place. When perceiving a stressor, such as experiencing negative emotions, self-regulating processes start by automatically activating the two main human stress mechanisms: the autonomic nervous system and the hypothalamic-pituitary-adrenal axis. Negative emotions are among the most important triggers of self-regulation failure.

Emotions regulation is the ability to manage one's emotions by the demands of the situation, is a skill that develops in early and middle childhood This skill is flexible and goal-directed, in that it is exercised when necessary to exhibit socially appropriate behaviors Therefore, emotion regulation manifests as situational-appropriate emotion expression, as one experiences an emotion and modulates its expression given the context.

Research regarding emotion regulation demonstrates this skill to be diagnostically relevant for child psychopathology. Children's feeling regulation difficulties, particularly with negative affect, are an established predictor of behavior problems and considered a risk factor for psychopathology. Some problems with emotion regulation can produce intense emotional expression, similar to the irritability present in ODD. For example, some ODD symptoms, such as bruxism, vindictiveness, and desire for revenge, contain emotional components and is the demonstration of strict emotion regulation strategies.

Researchers demonstrated that difficulties with anger regulation in preschooler kids were predictive of oppositional behaviors in elementary school. Children with and without behavior problems sometimes have the same peculiarities, even if there are a few differences. For instance, ODD children demonstrated more anger and impulsivity, as well as lower emotion regulation abilities, than children without behavioral difficulties

Another point of view is that children's reactivity may also contribute to their behavior problems That is, highly emotionally reactive kids, such as children with ODD, may need to engage in more emotion regulation strategies than other children to manage their intense feeling. In this sense, it is not that kids with ODD are not regulating their feelings but rather that it requires more emotion regulation to compensate for their high level of reactivity. So parents shape children's emotion regulation abilities through emotion socialization, in which they teach and demonstrate appropriate emotional expression.

In this way emotion socialization is a foundation for feeling Regulation Researchers suggest that children's emotion regulation deficits and consequent behavior problems also have origins in familiar approaches to children's emotions Known as emotion socialization, this is the process through which parents teach and model emotions for their children, as well as answer to their children's feelings.

Other psychologists analyze parental discussion of emotion and reactions to their children's feelings as two key emotion-related parenting practices that influence children's emotion regulation and therefore influence children's social behavior and social skill. In general, parental emotion-related discussion and reactions may either validate and encourage children's experience and appropriate expression of feelings, or dismiss and discourage children's experience and expression of emotions. Concluding a specific parental strategy, problem-solving about emotions, may be especially relevant for children with ODD because it models how to resolve distressing scenarios that may provoke negative consequences.

Emotion encouragement is theorized as parental acknowledgment and validation of children's feelings. This strategy is grounded in the belief that children's emotions have value and should be expressed. Many studies have demonstrated an association between emotion encouragement and emotion regulation in scholar kids. Some studies reported that familiar acceptance and support of emotional expression in fourth and fifth-grade children were linked to increased support seeking by children, one of the aforementioned emotion discouragement then, is characterized by parental disapproval of emotional expression. Parents who employ this strategy may be uncomfortable with emotions and thus seek to minimize or punish their children's emotions to decrease children's emotional expression.

Kid who receive punitive reactions for their emotions do not learn regulation strategies and therefore may experience more intense emotions. In a study of four to six-year-old typically developing children, researchers reported that mothers' unsupportive reactions to their children's negative emotions were related to children's difficulties regulating such effects.

So, parental minimization of children's emotions has also been associated with avoidant coping in third to sixth-grade kids. Although there are many studies of emotion discouragement in typically developing children, there is a lack of research regarding parental feelings of disappointment in families with atypically developing children. Some colleagues conducted a study, in which they examined kids five to eight years of age at risk for externalizing difficulties, such as ODD. They reported that parents' dismissal of children's emotions was linked with kids' difficulties with feelings regulation. Psychologists examined parental emotion discouragement in a sample of eight to twelve-year-old children with or without an anxiety disorder. Their findings indicate that mothers of anxious children spoke less than their children when discussing emotions, used fewer positive words, and discouraged emotions more than mothers of non-anxious kids. However, much remains to be discovered regarding parental emotion discouragement in children with oppositional behaviors and how this socialization strategy relates to children's emotion regulation.

ETIOLOGY AND RISK FACTORS

While no single cause of ODD has been identified, many risk factors and markers are associated with oppositional behavior.

Genetics

Genetic effects contribute significantly to the development of ODD symptoms with heritability estimates exceeding 50%, with genetic factors accounting for more than 70% of the variability in individual measures based on parent reports. While some have suggested that ODD shares substantial genetic overlap with conduct disorder, other studies have indicated unique effects for each. Also, it seems that genetic effects underlie the association between ODD and ADHD as well as between ODD and depressive disorder. In a twin study of adolescents, self-reported irritability symptoms of ODD "headstrong/hurtful" symptoms of ODD shared genetic risk with delinquent symptoms.

Age of onset

The age of onset of antisocial symptoms seems to be a good predictor of later outcomes. Researchers distinguish between children whose symptoms first emerge in childhood and persist into adolescence (childhood-onset persistent) compared to those whose symptoms first occur in adolescence. Individuals in the childhood-onset persistent group have been found to have poorer adult outcomes when compared with non-disordered and adolescent-onset peers.

Temperament

Temperamental factors in toddlerhood, such as irritability, impulsivity, and intensity of reactions to negative stimuli, may contribute to the development of a pattern of oppositional and defiant behavior. ODD may be arrived at through different temperamental routes that could serve to explain its comorbidity. The comorbidity between ODD and internalizing disorders is more strongly associated with early temperamental emotionality, whereas the comorbidity between ODD and ADDH is better predicted by temperamental overactivity.

Peer influences

Children who display oppositional behavior are more inclined to experience disrupted or problematic peer relationships. Such children are commonly rejected by non-deviant peers and tend instead to associate with other children who exhibit problem behavior. It would appear likely that the relationship between peer rejection and childhood ODD symptoms is a bi-directional one, as is nicely illustrated in a series of studies about bullying.

Callous and unemotional traits

The concept of psychopathy has been extended to young people in recent years with a focus on callous and unemotional traits. While not all children diagnosed with conduct disorder have callous and unemotional traits, the presence of such traits appears to distinguish a subgroup of children with more serious conduct problems. Callous and unemotional traits seem to be highly heritable and characterized by poor recognition of emotion (particularly fear) in facial expression.

Neighborhoods

The broader environment surrounding the child may also be a risk factor. Disruptive behavior has consistently been associated with social and economic disadvantage and neighborhood violence.

Family factors

The importance of the interplay between genes and family-level environmental factors has become increasingly clear in the etiology of children's disruptive behavior problems. Evidence from adoption studies shows that children at high genetic risk for antisocial behavior were more likely to receive negative parenting from the adoptive parents than were children with low genetic risk for antisocial behavior. Conversely, it is known from studies using a monozygotic twin design that family-level effects contribute to children's risk for externalizing problems over and above children's genetic effects. In other words, parental behavior towards children can be a true environmental risk.

Models of family influences

Parents of children with disruptive behavior problems are more likely to be inconsistent in how they apply rules, and give commands that are either unclear or the result of their own current emotional state rather than contingent upon the child's behavior. A typical mutually coercive process would arise when a parent responds in an unduly harsh way to a child's mildly disruptive behavior, upon which the child may further escalate its oppositional behavior. This in turn leads to yet harsher responses by the parent with further escalation. The result is that the parent may in the end give in, reinforcing the child's negative behaviors. This paradoxical "reward" of a child's negative behavior may both increase and maintain oppositional behaviors and is the specific target of therapeutic interventions.

ODD within the School Setting

Children with the ODD diagnosis struggle in the school setting, but the school setting allows for early intervention and provides an opportunity for an all-around team treatment approach. Between 10 and 12 percent of children experience moderately clinical problems during their school careers; many of these children are oppositionally defiant to authority and predisposed to conduct disorder in the absence of intervention. When treating a child who has ODD, like many other diagnoses, early intervention is key.

Although ODD is typically diagnosed at a later age, the school can provide an environment for early treatment approaches at the first sign of potential behavior problems. Often if children with ODD go undiagnosed and untreated, the oppositional behavior in adolescence can lead to other disorders such as conduct disorder. The school provides an environment for early treatment approaches to begin within the preschool setting starting at age four. In some cases, successful intervention can begin even earlier at 12 months of age up to 6 years old. Further, early intervention even in early elementary school years can significantly decrease future behavioral disorders in later life. Along with early intervention, school-based interventions for children with ODD need to include a comprehensive approach where one includes all systems of the child, including family, school staff, and community service providers. Many times providers work on various treatment methods independently and are not using the same interventions across multiple settings. As is, little programming is created for school-age children that have ODD where the family is treated as a system and is involved in the treatment.

However, if the child's mental health treatment provider can be responsible for bringing the interventions to the school setting and home setting, the child's behavior will improve. This consistency in the home environment and the school environment allows for children to thrive and gain a sense of independence. Not only is treatment important to establish across all settings, but diagnosing needs to be done comprehensively as well. A child with ODD will demonstrate oppositional behavior at home and school. Providing intervention to one half of the environment will not fix the problem.

Family Approach to School-Based Intervention

For children to be successful within the school setting, the family needs to be involved with treatment. The school environment allows for families to be involved in treatment, mental health providers within the school to work within the school and home environments, and consistency across settings.

Parenting is a major development in changing aggressive and oppositional behavior within the school setting. To be successful in the school environment, treatment on the home front is crucial. Many times schools do not include parents with the intervention that is being utilized with their child. However, the school is the environment where family-centered approaches to interventions can be successful. This team approach can start with the formation of an Individualized Education Plan (IEP).

In 1975 Public Law 94-142 was established and the IEP was born. The IEP gives an education plan that is specific to that child that receives special education including the children with externalizing disorders such as ODD. The IEP document provides compliance, services, and guidelines for children who have physical, mental, and learning disabilities in the school setting and provides them with adequate educational opportunities. There is no document more significant to districts, agencies, administrators, teachers, parent and educational advocates, and students. With the IEP signatures and meetings are scheduled at least yearly to meet the needs of the children. In school-based intervention, the IEP is the start of the involvement with the parents. Further, mental health providers in the school can be contacted before, during, or after these meetings and conferences occur, allowing for easy access to mental health treatment. At this point, the mental health treatment can be accessed across all settings, home and school, to provide a consistent treatment approach.

Treatment Approaches to Oppositional Defiant Disorder

Family-centered school-based interventions for treating children with oppositional defiant disorder should include social-learning family interventions (SLFI). SLFI approaches are the most successful when treating children with externalizing behavioral disorders. Researchers go on to discuss 4 steps for families to treat non-compliant children with the SLFI approach by first, "watching the child's play rather than direct it" and then "engaging in the activities". The second step is for parents to "reinforce positive behavior in social situations." The third step is for parents to "state commands simply." The final step is for parents to "learn to use time-outs for non-compliant behavior.". Two different SLFI approaches that can be successful family-centered school-based interventions within the school setting are Incredible Years training and Tuesday's Child training.

Incredible Years training seeks to prevent children with behavioral disorders, such as ODD, to continue as disruptive in late elementary and within adolescence. Incredible Years implements this intervention by using interactional parenting models to enhance a child's well being. These interactional parenting models can be learned through role-play, videos, and group parenting sessions. Further, the school can adapt these models and utilize them in the classroom setting as well, to be consistent in treatment. A study done using Incredible Years training on Portuguese families in the school setting yielded positive results on parent/teacher-child interactions and improved the child's oppositional behavior.

A second SLFI approach that can be modeled as a family-centered intervention within the school setting is the Tuesday's Child approach. Tuesday's Child approach emphasizes the importance of family-centered practice in five ways. First, there are structured ways in teaching parents how to effectively intervene with their oppositional child, thus making the parent feel empowered. The second way is assessing with a mental health professional and using individualized treatment methods to meet the individualized need of the child in the home and school settings. The third way family-centered practice is emphasized is that the families meet at the school for treatment, which allows school staff and practitioners to reach the family and child in a safe environment. Fourth, the social work systems approach is being utilized. The parents, services, and school are looked at as systems that need to be adjusted, providing a consistent structure for the child. Fifth, within the systems method, a team approach is being yielded, where the different service providers can discuss interventions with each other. The Tuesday's Child approach may create the tools necessary for the parent and school to be successful in creating a positive environment for the child to grow and cope positively. Another form of intervention that can be used within the school setting is understanding the temperament qualities of students with ODD to further assess the student's strengths and weaknesses. When looking at a temperament dimension there is a strong side and an "underdeveloped" side which leads to negative behaviors.

    They propose that when a teacher or professional has an understanding of their strong attributes they can successfully use those attributes when working with those children. When looking at the extroverted-introverted styles, a child with ODD has extraverted qualities. The strengths of extraverted qualities include "enjoying group discussions, a wide range of topic interests, and a preference for verbal responses". Another temperament trait identified is the practical-imaginative style. Children with ODD are practical in that they "have rigid attitudes, narrow focus on present issues, and failure to consider long-term consequences for behaviors". It is noted that for students with a practical orientation, such as children with ODD, providing very specific rules in every situation and discussing the consequence of each rule can be beneficial in changing defiant behavior. A third temperament to be discussed is the thinking-feeling style. Children with ODD to have a Thinking style due to "blunt verbal interactions and initiate debate in provoking or responding to conflict". Children with ODD often fail to seek harmony and closure, and would rather confront conflict, demonstrating the Thinking preference.

Children with ODD demonstrate a flexible temperament style whose weakness is organizational skills and compliance. Children with ODD are more apt to display minimal self-control and little compliance to the classroom structure. This can be demonstrated in the behavior of "losing their temper, blame others for misfortunes, argue, defy rules, and neglect to follow procedures". If the temperament styles of a child with ODD are identified, the teacher, professional, and parent would be able to plan interventions accordingly. Knowing the temperament of a child allows those to pursue the child's strengths and build those strengths through positive interventions. For a child diagnosed with ODD to be successful within the school setting, all systems need to be involved in a comprehensive treatment approach. It is unclear how these interventions and other interventions are being used within the school setting. This study looks to explore treatment models that can be used within the school setting for children to answer the question: What school-based interventions are effective in school settings for students who are diagnosed with Oppositional Defiant Disorder?

There is no one-size-fits-all treatment for children and adolescents with ODD. The most effective treatment plans are tailored to the needs and behavioral symptoms of each child. Treatment decisions are typically based on several different things, including the child's age, the severity of the behaviors, and whether the child has a coexisting mental health condition.

The goals and circumstances of the parents also are important when forming a treatment plan. In different cases, treatment may last several months or years and requires commitment and follow-through by parents as well as by others involved in the child's care.

Different types of treatment usually consists of a combination of: Parent-Management Training Programs and Family Therapy to teach parents and other family members how to manage the child's behavior. These techniques are a positive reinforcement and a way to discipline more effectively.

Another important key could be the use of cognitive Problem-Solving Skills Training to reduce inappropriate behaviors by teaching the child or the teenager positive ways of responding to stressful situations. Children and teenagers with ODD only know of negative ways of responding to real-life situations. Social-Skills Programs and School-Based Programs to teach children and adolescents how to relate more positively to others and ways to improve their school work.

These therapies are successfulwhen they are settled in a natural environment, such as at the school or in a social group. Sometimes medication may be necessary to help control some of the more distressing symptoms of ODD as well as the symptoms of coexisting conditions, such as ADHD, anxiety, and mood disorders. However, medication alone is not a complete treatment for defiant children.

For preschool-age children, treatment often concentrates on parent-management training and education. School-age children perform best with a combination of school-based intervention, parent management training, and individual therapy. For adolescents, individual therapy along with parent-management training is the most effective form of treatment.

Parent-Management Training Studies have shown that intervening with parents is one of the most effective ways to reduce the behavioral symptoms of defiant children in all age groups. Parent management training teaches parents positive ways to manage their child's behavior, discipline techniques, and age-appropriate supervision. It is the treatment of choice to prevent disruptive childhood behavior for many mental health professionals.

This approach embraces the following principles:
- Increased positive parenting practices, such as providing supportive and consistent supervision and discipline

- Decreased negative parenting practices, such as the use of harsh punishment and focus on inappropriate behaviors
- Consistent punishment for disruptive behavior
- Predictable, immediate parental response

Sex differences in oppositional defiant disorder

Various studies have shown that the prevalence of ODD is greater in boys than in girls. However, questions have arisen over whether this difference is real, or an effect of the way the disorder is defined. In the last ten years, there has been a debate over whether it is appropriate to use common diagnostic criteria for boys and girls in externalizing disorders such as ODD. Girls' aggressiveness is manifested in covert, less observable ways, to exclude peers, whilst boys' aggressive behaviors are more obvious and have been associated with deficits in moral processing. There may be a sample of girls with behavior problems, with greater impairment in their level of functioning than the girls in their normative group, and whom the current diagnostic criteria fail to identify. The definition of ODD include relational aggression behaviors (refusing to talk to someone, being malicious, avoiding blame) in the identification of girls with oppositional characteristics.

The fact that the tendency to present oppositional behaviors and disruptive emotions (anger, poking fun, etc.) is more commonly observed in boys than in girls is consistent with the theory that the expression of anger is more common and acceptable in boys, which may explain, in part, the greater presence of externalizing problems in boys. However, in clinical samples, ODD is also associated with anxiety disorders. ODD may be a precursor of anxiety problems in the future. In children with higher levels of anxiety, this anxiety was often manifested through oppositional behavior.

Although there is evidence of comorbidity between ODD and internalizing disorders, it is not clear whether this association is stronger in boys or girls. Sex differences in the comorbidity of oppositional behavior, both with other externalizing disorders and with internalizing disorders, imply different biological and socialization factors. Studies on role expectations according to sex have shown that boys learn that anger and aggression are more acceptable emotions in males than anxiety, sadness or fear, and that they are reinforced more in boys than in girls. Such subtle socialization styles may contribute to differences between sexes in internalizing symptoms and in externalizing behaviors. Given that anxiety is more common among girls and oppositional behavior is more common in boys, but at the same time anxiety and oppositional behavior are also correlated with one another, it is important to ascertain whether greater comorbidity is associated with sex. The association between oppositional behavior and daily functioning difficulties has been less studied. The degree to which a particular disorder interferes with or impairs an individual's everyday life is one of the most relevant variables for reaching a diagnosis, and for establishing the need for intervention.

Age differences in oppositional defiant disorder

Unlike adults, children are rapidly and constantly changing both physically and psychologically. As children grow and change, it is natural for them to go through periods of rebelliousness and opposition to authority. Children are expected to display labile moods, hostility, and attempts to flout the control of authorities, particularly during those times known as the terrible twos and adolescence. Research has shown that children as young as 3 or 4 can have externalizing problems that are abnormal for their age. The fact that children as young as 3 or 4 can present abnormal opposition and conduct problems reveal the importance of understanding the unique presentation of these behaviors at various ages, and that these unique presentations should be accounted for in future criteria for ODD.

However, 3 and 4-year-olds with externalizing behavior problems are not going to present with the same issues as 10-year-olds. Neither will 11-year-olds and 17-year-olds going to present with the same issues. The severity of impairment based on the same behavior at various ages may also be an important factor. For example a 4-9-year-old who purposely engages in actions that could result in serious injury to another person may represent a more severe level of impairment than the same act committed by a 14-17-year-old who has easier access and more ability to commit the act, as well as knowledge of the real consequences of hurting someone else. Discovering how ODD is displayed by specific age groups should be an important area of research in the future, and an issue for clinicians to be aware of when assessing ODD in youth.

It is thought that these children progress from relatively less serious forms of [Conduct Problems] (e.g., noncompliance, temper tantrums) to more serious forms (e.g., aggression, stealing, substance abuse) over time, that more overt behaviors (e.g., defiance, fighting) appear earlier than covert behaviors (those that occur behind the backs of adult caregivers, such as lying and stealing), and that later [Conduct Problems] expand the child's behavioral repertoire rather than replace earlier behaviors. Furthermore, there is an expansion of the settings in which the [Conduct Problems] occur over time, from the home to other settings such as the school and the broader community.

Culture differences in oppositional defiant disorder

Different cultures can have highly contrasting expectations of children depending on the sex or age of the child. For example, many religiously conservative families expect their daughters to stay at home and raise children rather than continuing with further education or careers. Even different generations can add complexity to the situation. For example, a young child's liberal and permissive parents die, and the child is suddenly placed with his/her grandparents who use a more conservative and authoritarian style the child is not used to. A study found that the prevalence of ODD remained similar despite the content of the study (primarily North America and Europe). However, some data appears to confirm that cultural perceptions of the role of girls in society play a role in the rates of ODD.

Oppositional Defiant Disorder in Adolescents

Adolescence is a stage of life that results in many changes. Some of these changes are biological such as a time of rapid growth in height, weight, and sexual maturation. These biological changes can influence social and emotional changes as well. In some cases, teens become more self-conscious and concerned with their peer groups which replace their families as being central in their lives. Risk-taking behaviors can increase, and interests can change. Because of these changes and other factors in their lives, middle school can be a challenging time for students.

When people ask about the career of this researcher and are told she is a middle school teacher and attends graduate school to become a school counselor, the typical reactions include: "Oh, you must be an angel!", or "I could never do that!", and "Kids that age are so disrespectful! " While occasionally in agreement with the thought expressed by others, working with middle-school-age adolescents is very rewarding. Yes, there are some difficult students and difficult situations, but the "tough" or "disrespectful" children in this age group are not the only kids in the middle schools, and helping them is just as rewarding as helping the other students who are not quite as outwardly "tough." Some of the children who appear to have more challenges and who are tougher and more disrespectful to authority are sometimes diagnosed with Oppositional Defiant Disorder.

It is important to talk to the child first and not jump directly to punishment. Set the stage for the conversation by letting the child know in advance that good listening is important and "if he or she fails to listen and make good decisions, then immediate consequences will follow". The conversation is not to convince the child to agree with the parent, and should not be stated this way. Instead, a brief, straightforward statement of intent is best. Follow-through is essential. Good discipline includes one-on-one conversations that begin with a tone and posture that are friendly but firm to establish the roles of adult and child. Adolescents need to understand that their actions impact others and if the behavior is negative, adults need to explain why behavior needs to change. Consequences and replacement behaviors need to be clearly stated and understood. Replacement thoughts are also helpful to deter inappropriate future behavior. All behaviors have positive and negative consequences.

Oppositional defiant adolescents do not always foresee the potential negative consequences of their actions. As a result, the negative consequence needs to be stronger than what the adolescent sees as positive reinforcement of the behavior. "Oppositional defiant and conduct-disordered adolescents have tremendous difficulty accepting limits. They routinely stretch rules and react negatively to any imposition of authority. Their lack of self-control fuels much of their deviant behavior.

Setting limits and following-through with enforcement can help by protecting the adolescents and others from their impulsive nature. Parents, teachers, and counselors need to monitor and anticipate the need for such limits and be firm with them. Signs of ODD. may include escalating emotions, hyper-reactivity, and defensive posturing were responding to and diffusing the situation externally would be necessary. Limits can be discussed with the adolescents by reasoning that the more control they have on their actions and the more responsibility they take for their behavior, the lesser the need for external control or limits imposed by others. Pointing out the choices in the situation and listening for cues that the adolescents sometimes give to invite adults to set limits for them is often helpful. There are indications that children who are temperamentally difficult from birth who receive positive parenting avoid becoming more oppositional. However, children who are treated negatively with harsh discipline or inconsistency, often become more disruptive and harder to handle as they get older.

Education is the key and being informed is the first step that school counselors need to take to help students with Oppositional Defiant Disorder, their parents, and other school personnel. Since school counselors are an integral part of children's support system, counselors are often some of the first to intervene with children with ODD when they are disruptive or have inappropriate behavior in schools. One of the first steps counselors should take to help a child with ODD. is talking with the parents, teachers, and child to find out what triggers the child's feelings that may lead to defiant behavior. Next, the counselor would make observations in the classroom and other areas of the school such as the lunchroom and playground to note the interaction the student has with others. It is crucial to understand as much as possible about the child and determine what triggers the feelings, and what motivates his or her behavior.

School counselors can help students by providing anger management and social relationship skills to small groups of students or with individual students. Problem-solving and communication skills are two more themes that can be beneficial to work on with a child with ODD.

Children with ODD often misinterpret social cues and have trouble appropriately expressing their negative feelings, so learning about what triggers the defiant feelings, identifying them themselves, and then reacting appropriately are the first steps. "If children become more tuned into their body signals, they can take care of themselves and deal with the anger and the precipitant for their anger before they blow". Relaxation training may lower the child's tension level so that he can think more clearly and have less reactive behavior. This may help children assertively communicate their feelings and needs without anger getting in the way of their messages. They are taught to solve problems in a different way than they have done in the past, which can be more effective with a relaxed, clearheaded approach.

School counselors can also be resources for overwhelmed teachers who work with children with ODD. For example, counselors can be helpful when unsafe conditions are created in the school or classroom or when the teacher needs help coping with the stress of teaching defiant and uncooperative children in the classroom. A very important point about working with adolescents who have ODD is: "the dominant thoughts of the oppositional child revolve around defeating anyone's attempt to exercise authority over him". Keeping this in mind, researchers listed rules or guidelines to help people such as parents, teachers, and school counselors who work with and care for children with ODD. For example, oppositional children seem to live in a fantasy land where they can defeat all authority figures. In this way, they are optimistic, yet may fail to learn from experience. Oppositional children believe, "You must be fair to me, regardless of how I treat you," and then often seek revenge when things do not go their way. They have a need to feel tough, and if they ignore authority long enough, eventually the person will give up and go away as they feel equal with adults in power. Oppositional children from middle-class homes often emulate the behavior of their least-successful peers. Oppositional children and teenagers attempt to answer most questions with "I don't know" and deny responsibility. Replacement thoughts can help by taking the place of the perceptions that seem to dominate the thinking of adolescents with ODD.

For example, rather than thinking that they can defeat all adults, keeping in mind that adults own everything and can take it away if they choose, may change a teen's thinking. Also, revenge is not always the best option. For teens who think it is, a visit to people in prison to ask them how well their revenge strategies worked may prove them wrong.

Follow-through is essential, so if consequences are stated, it is important to ensure that they happen. Caring adults choose their battles when dealing with, teaching, or counseling children who are controlling and defiant. Attention-getting clothing, style of appearance, use of jargon or profanity, or other actions that initiate annoyances may be used to test limits and reactions. Unless extreme, adults would do well simply to ignore such behaviors as conveying clear expectations kids learn they can control their actions without much adult intervention. It is important to demonstrate that adults are neither intimidated nor compelled to discipline them for minor infractions.

When this strategy is practiced, most find that the provocative behavior dissipates rapidly, that is, the teen will put down the rubber band or simply pick up the trash that has missed the wastebasket. Moreover, oppositional defiant youth are instinctively defensive as "They have great difficulty accepting any confrontation that could perforate their defensive structure". Their appearances are very important to note, and that while the adolescents may not tell the whole truth, their appearance often will. Gently pointing out discrepancies between their words and appearances or body language can be helpful and help them to open up. Over time, as relationships are established and the child learns to trust, his or her self-awareness increases.

To work effectively with adolescents with Oppositional Defiant Disorder, the definition of oppositional behavior must be clearly understood by all who are working with the adolescents so everyone is on the same page. Forming a partnership with the child, the parents, and the school can create the needed structure the child needs. This partnership and understanding can lead to interventions and strategies to help the student find opportunities to become successful in the home and school.

Parental approach

In this chapter, you will understand what you can do as a parent, while in the next chapter I will give guidance on what to do as a teacher. Now it's useful to step back to our possible "prejudices" about ADHD, ODD or defiant children, which can affect working with the child. This, in other words, means that how each one approaches the problem is not trivial; on the contrary, it confirms that it is important that you become aware of the more or less clear perception that you have of the disorder and of the situation you are experiencing.

To achieve this awareness, it is important to reflect on the idea you have of your child; for this reason, while before focusing our attention on general aspects of the disorder, now it's better to induce reflection on what each one thinks of their child, in particular.

The premise is that all of us when we live something, when we have a success or a failure, we need to give us an explanation of what happened to us because things went just that way. Psychologists speak of attributive style because in some way the person needs to attribute what happened to one cause rather than another.

The attributive style in generic terms can be external or internal: that is, so we can think that things have gone a certain way or because have been, if successful, lucky or because you are intelligent and able to manage them in a certain way. In the first case using an external style, that is, do not recognize the responsibility for what you have done, it depends on an external factor. If, on the other hand, you are using an internal style, It's recognizable that in some way you play an important role in what is happening around you, in my successes or my failures. It may seem strange to us, but that's exactly how we work, and the prediction we make about a certain event greatly influences the success of a certain situation and possibly its resolution.

And at this point, we can tell a story about the power of thought. For years it was believed impossible for athletes to be able to run a mile within 4 minutes: in all the races in the world, the champions were unable to improve this time. Then a British athlete, Roger Bannister, in 1954, conquered the record of a mile in less than 4 min.

The belief of succeeding has contributed, in the case of this athlete, to the modification of behavior!

Advice for parenting ODD

Relating to an ODD kid is difficult and complicated and sometimes you can easily lose your temper for his/her unpredictable actions or answers. Here for you a guideline to better manage your relationship, and some advice you can adopt in different occasions. Defiant children usually escalate to violence and this is a bad symptom that could end in a social maladjustment. The first thing you should do is accepting your kid's problem and change your mindset about it. Punishment is never educative and in this case could hurt and make things worst, because punishment it's not efficient in these cases.

- Understand that your child has a problem and admit it to yourself.
- Try to build a strong relationship with your kid and effort it with time spent together. For instance, you could build something or paint, everything creative is relaxing, and do it every day. Listen to what he/she likes, doing things together effort positively your relationship.

- Try to be patient and compassionable, not too strict, understand that your kid it's impulsive and sensitive at the same time.
- Model your own emotions and reactions, trying to answer with calm, breath ...everything it's ok. Your kid should always relate with someone confident, so try to be self-confident above all.
- Be responsible for your emotions controlling your sensitiveness, even when he/she loses temper.
- Abolish any form of aggression, screaming wouldn't help you.
- Work together in a team, educate him/her to action consequences and dissimulate when you are in public and she/he is very nervous or anxious.
- Using code words could help you to manage your relationship and their moment of stress. Instead of NO or Enough or even Stop, choose together a special word as Chocolate or Candy to evidence something is not going in the right way, he/she is screaming or losing temper.
- Your child should know who makes the rules... You! So be clear about it.

- Breath and count till 10 every time you have to answer to his/her crisis.
- Call a professional psychologist and think about using medications. Is your kid's reaction reasonable? And is his/her behavior proper? Sometimes you can't make it on your own.
- PARENTAL PROBLEM SOLVING (you are the one supposed to solve any situation so b responsible and conscious!)

A crisis occurs any time that your child is no longer safe to himself or others or when there is a need for immediate action or intervention. It is usually a moment when all of your energies are being demanded to care for your child.

Diet

Child behavior and food are closely linked. Studies show that certain foods can cause or at least worsen behavioral issues like ADHD and other learning disorders.

Some of the common foods that can cause ODD reactions include milk, chocolate, soy, wheat, eggs, beans, corn, tomatoes, grapes, and oranges, and of course coffee. If you suspect a food sensitivity may be contributing to your child's ODD symptoms, talk to your dietitian or doctor about trying an elimination.

If you suspect something in his/her diet could increase these ODD behave, you can ask your doctor and exclude little by little some food you are suspicious of. According to many nutrition experts, the top common food intolerances include:

- milk or cheese
- eggs
- gluten - Protein in Wheat, Rye, Oats, and Barley
- sugar (Particularly if your child has candida, a yeast overgrowth that can affect behavior,

common in children with neuro-behavioral disorders like ADHD and Autism.)
- Shellfish
- Soy
- Foods High in Salicylate and salt
- Food Dyes, Preservatives, Pesticides, GMO's food in general.

The link between diet and behavior is an interesting one, especially when food sensitivities are involved. If a child is intolerant to a particular food, a reaction occurs. This reaction stems from the immune system and causes the body to produce inflammatory chemicals called cytokines. Cytokines can inflame the gut, brain, or respiratory tract and ultimately affect how your child feels physically and emotionally. A healthful diet may reduce symptoms by reducing exposure and additives and improving the intake of omega-3 fats and micro-nutrients. But it certainly will improve overall health and nutrition, and set the stage for a lifetime of good health.

Parental Problem solving to manage ODD.

The most important peculiarity parents should practice is problem-solving, especially in the case of ODD. Problem-solving is a process through which families aid their kids in identifying causes, consequences, and future solutions to emotion eliciting situations. Problem-solving can be theorized as an emotion socialization strategy, in that the parent is teaching the child appropriate ways to handle emotionally laden situations.

Anyway, this strategy is distinct from emotion encouragement and discouragement because it concerns discussion of the situation rather than validating or dismissing the emotion itself. Given that problem solving is a strategy to modulate effect, assisting the kid in knowing the problem and developing strategies for future situations, this can be understood as a model of appropriate behaviors and thus indicative of children's.

Feelings regulation skills. These connections have been supported in helping kids developing, though associations differ by parent and child gender. reported that maternal problem-focused coping was associated with adaptive coping in third to sixth-grade children, where this link was not present with fathers. other, parental problem-focused coping has also been linked with modulated effect in first to fourth-grade boys, but not girls Concerning atypically developing children, there is little research regarding parental problem solving as a strategy to foster children's emotion regulation, as it is often incorporated as a composite of supportive parenting researchers studied nine to thirteen-year-old African American kids living in violent cities contexts, a risk factor for ODD.

Observations of mother-child conversations of feelings indicated that maternal problem-solving suggestions were associated with children's problem-focused coping. However, much is still to be discovered, as the majority of research regarding problem-solving strategies and atypically developing children pertains to the effectiveness of problem-solving interventions for children with behavior problems, rather than parent problem-solving strategies.

ODD, autism, and ADHD

Children with ODD and conduct disorder are characterized by persistent antisocial and aggressive behaviors. Kids suffering from ODD and CD are at risk for numerous negative outcomes, such as violence, unemployment, depression, anxiety, and other psychiatric problems. Recognizing risk factors for antisocial and aggressive behavior that can be targeted for potential change is very important. Lately, it has been showing that problems in feeling regulation, referring to the processes by which individuals influence which emotions they have, when they have them, and how they experience and express this emotion may be an important mechanism driving behavioral problems in ODD.

Defective emotion regulation skills are also thought to drive behavior problems in kids with other psychiatric disorders, such as autism spectrum disorders and attention-deficit/hyperactivity disorder ADHD. Therefore, there is a need to investigate if emotion regulation difficulties exist in those with ODD/CD, and to what extent emotion regulation difficulties are related to comorbid autism and attention deficit traits in those with ODD/CD, using cognitive, behavioral, and self-report measures of emotion regulation. emotion regulation is necessary for psychological well-being and social functioning. Although emotion regulation strategies can be used deliberately, often these processes operate unconsciously. In real life, we are regularly confronted with situations eliciting emotions. Feeling regulation helps us to answer to those emotions in a socially acceptable and flexible way.

Impaired emotion regulation abilities in children have been associated with reduced prosocial behavior and increased vulnerability for psychopathology. Researchers showed that there are several empirical studies in support of the hypothesis that emotion regulation may be compromised in children with aggressive and antisocial behavior. Effective emotion regulation starts with emotional awareness, defined as attention to and insight into one's emotional responses and functioning. Incomplete emotional consciousness may lead to handling unpleasant emotions with impulsive acting-out behavior, because of misinterpreted internal and external emotional cues.

Children with aggression problems are less likely to inhibit emotional reactivity and used less effective or more inappropriate regulatory strategies, thus emotion dysregulation is a strong predictor of aggressive behavior in an adolescent community sample and not vice versa. Emotion dysregulation is not specific for children with ODD/CD. Children with other psychiatric disorders, such as ADHD or ASD, also have emotion regulation difficulties Symptoms rates of ODD or CD in children with ADHD is high, more than 59%. Aggression is displayed in over 50% of the children with ASD.

Children with ADHD lack the capacity for inhibition, making it difficult for them to delay a response long enough to gather information necessary for understanding emotionally charged situations. Children with ASD are prone to react impulsively to emotional stimuli with tantrums, aggression, or self-injury, which is thought to result from impaired emotion regulation abilities. Now thanks to modern researches we all know that ADHD is associated with emotional dysregulation only in the presence of a comorbid disorder, such as ODD, anxiety or depression, or CD.

Conclusions

Odd kids have a lot of difficulties to express their emotions and problems in understanding their feelings. Parents should always be able to manage this behavior and when is necessary ask for external help or think about medications. Families need as the most important ability "problem solving" that is useful especially in public. Odd is not always recognizable, even if some aspects are useful to predict this defiant behavior. Researches demonstrate that how parents discuss feelings with their children and react to children's emotions is indicative of children's ability to modulate their emotional experience and expression.

This link is very important to consider during middle childhood, at which point children begin to independently manage their emotions. Janitorial responses that encourage children to express feelings and develop solutions for their emotional distress may foster children's skills to handle intense feelings experiences. On the contrary, punitive and dismissive responses to children's emotions may not provide kids with knowledge of adaptive regular abilities. It is important to note that children's emotion regulation abilities may also influence parent's socialization strategies.

Highly reactive children, such as children with ODD, may stand to receive a greater benefit from parent feeling socialization as they may need to implement more emotion regulation strategies to behave in a socially appropriate manner. By the same token, they may also be more vulnerable to the negatives effects associated with minimizing and punitive socialization strategies, as this may lead to deficits in what are already insufficient emotion regulation skills.

CPSIA information can be obtained
at www.ICGtesting.com
Printed in the USA
LVHW080506290521
688869LV00009B/593